PERIMENOPAUSE GUIDE FOR WOMEN

A Comprehensive Handbook from Perimenopause to Postmenopausal Wisdom

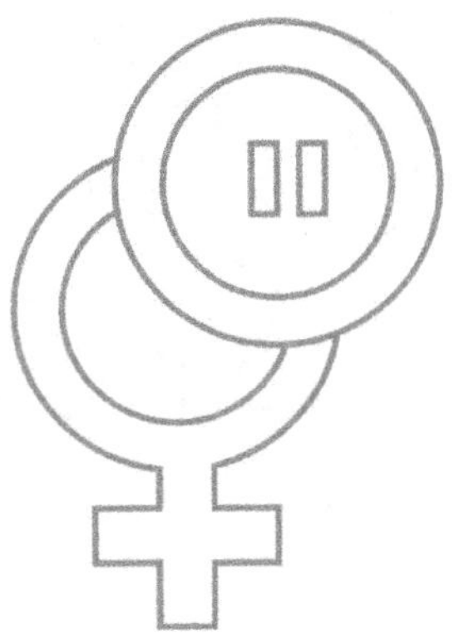

SAVANNAH USHER

TABLE OF CONTENTS

Introduction

Perimenopause is a crucial and transforming chapter in the broad scheme of a woman's life, bringing with it a symphony of changes that can be both thrilling and difficult. This is the " Perimenopause Guide for Women." Welcome to its pages. Perimenopause is without a doubt one of the most fascinating and complex plot twists in literature about life.

Let's embrace the natural progression of perimenopause as we set out on this adventure together. Perimenopause is a time when the body performs a symphony of hormonal changes that cause a variety of physical, emotional, and mental upheavals. This compassionately produced guide is meant to be a kind companion that will illuminate your path through this remarkable stage of life.

We'll explore the perimenopause's complexities in these pages, demystifying its subtleties and arming you with information. Think of this manual as a compass that will lead you through the unknown world of mood swings, hormone changes, and bodily metamorphoses. Not only do we want to educate you, but we also want to travel with you, providing support and friendship along the route.

The perimenopause is like a soft murmur, signaling changes that could start off as a mild wind and intensify over time into a fierce storm. We will examine the intricacies of these modifications, identifying the preliminary indications of perimenopausal symptoms. Together, we'll explore the basic foundations and comprehend the hormonal dance that affects your body, mind, and soul.

Perimenopause is an emotional roller coaster that goes beyond the physical changes. It's a period of self-discovery during which time familiar landscapes could take on new colors and your identity's shapes might change. We'll take a deep dive into emotional health, covering anxiety, mood swings, and all the emotions that come with going through this life-changing stage.

But worry not—this guide is more than just a wayfinding aid for obstacles. It also honors resiliency and self-determination. We'll look at ways to control physical health through good sleep hygiene, exercise regimens, and dietary knowledge. We will talk about developing closeness and effective communication techniques as relationships traverse the ups and downs of hormonal waves.

The subject of hormone replacement therapy (HRT) comes up frequently when people talk about perimenopause. We'll dissect the subtleties of HRT in these pages, offering a fair assessment of its benefits and drawbacks to enable you to make wise decisions regarding your health.

However, our voyage goes beyond traditional methods. As we explore integrative medicine, herbal cures, and mind-body activities that align with your body's natural cycles, holistic well-being takes center stage. It's about adopting a holistic strategy for wellness that fits your particular path.

And when we finally round the corner, we'll look toward the menopause, explaining the shift and joyfully welcoming the years that follow perimenopause. Perimenopause is a chapter that enhances the story of your life, which is one of development, resiliency, and strength.

So keep in mind that you're not alone as you begin this journey, dear reader. This book is your warm, wise, and supportive travel companion through the complex and breathtaking terrain of the perimenopause. Together, let's set out on this adventure to uncover the beauty and strength that are inside each of you.

CHAPTER 1: Understanding Perimenopause

Introduction to Perimenopause

Ahh, the perimenopause, that delicate yet potent shift that signifies a major turning point in the life of every woman. It's similar to setting foot on undiscovered territory when your body, mind, and emotions undergo a metamorphosis. Imagine it as a slowly flowing stream of change, frequently accompanied by waves of exploration and the sporadic unpredictability of a storm. But, have no fear—this is a normal aspect of being a woman and a stage that bridges the gap between your impressionable youth and mature understanding.

Before delving into the complex picture of perimenopause, let's clarify the purpose of this trip. Often called the forerunner to menopause, perimenopause usually begins in a woman's forties, though others may experience it earlier or later. Hormonal swings and the body's preparation for the end of the menstrual cycle interact delicately.

Let's talk about hormones now, the orchestra conductors of this composition. Progesterone and the charismatic lead, estrogen, bow down politely to each other. These hormonal dynamics set off a series of physiological changes in your body, much like a delicate dance. Even if this sounds like a complicated dance routine, it's important to understand that these changes are just as normal as the tides coming in and going out.

You may notice unusual patterns in your menstrual cycle during the early stages of perimenopause. If your monthly visitor shows up out of the blue or takes a little break, don't be alarmed. All it is is your body getting used to a new rhythm. Additionally, hot flashes—those impulsive bursts of warmth—may appear. Think of them as the body's signal that "Change is in the air!"

However, perimenopause has a way of accessing your emotional reserves in addition to physical changes. Mood fluctuations could intensify and resemble the shifting colors of a sunset. You may experience a sudden rush of sadness or be overcome with a sense of contentment. It's completely natural, and accepting these feelings as a necessary component of your own path can feel incredibly freeing.

Consider the perimenopause as a starting point for personal growth. It's a chance to take stock of your life and make it fresh and imaginative. These changes in your body are an invitation to explore the depth of your resilience, to connect with your inner self, and to develop a fresh respect for the woman you are becoming.

Recognizing the variety of perimenopausal feelings is crucial. Some people might have little trouble making this change, while others might find it a little more difficult. Recognize that you are not alone on any road you choose. Generations of women have navigated this terrain together as a sisterhood, providing a wealth of experience, knowledge, and support.

So let's approach this research of perimenopause with inquiry and friendship, my dear friend. Consider it an adventure, an opportunity to navigate unknown waters with the wind of self-discovery guiding you. Together, we will solve the puzzles of perimenopause while providing support, comfort, and a helping hand.

Prepare yourself for the journey that lies ahead: a journey across the oceans of change, where every wave has the possibility of revealing renewed fortitude, resiliency, and the beauty of accepting life's inevitable changes. Let the journey begin - welcome to the perimenopause!

The Biological Basis

The perimenopause is an intriguing time when a woman's biology undergoes a complex and distinct transformation. Knowing the facts behind this transforming phase's biological underpinnings is not as important as developing a deeply personal connection with your body.

Hormone dances delicately at the center of perimenopause. Think of your reproductive system as an orchestra, with progesterone and estrogen playing lead roles and directing the music. Now, this symphony changes in subtle yet profound ways as you get closer to this stage of life.

Known as the "queen of hormones," estrogen fluctuates during the perimenopause. Once steady, its levels now begin a rhythmic dance, getting your body ready for the next big act in the magnificent show of womanhood. The emotional and physical changes that accompany perimenopause are mostly brought on by these fluctuations in hormone levels.

Progesterone, estrogen's faithful companion, should also not be overlooked. Over the years, they have collaborated to plan your menstrual cycles. However, progesterone's function changes when the perimenopause takes center stage. Its levels could drop, which would affect the entire hormonal tapestry and cause variations in your menstrual cycle.

The ovaries, those inconspicuous builders of fertility, likewise alter when these hormonal changes take place. The ovarian reserve, which was formerly abundant in eggs, eventually runs out. Consider it to be nature's gentle way of ushering you into the next phase of your life after motherhood. It's a normal course of events, a steady pulse in the aging symphony.

During perimenopause, the menstrual cycle, a monthly pattern that has followed you since youth, becomes a little more erratic. The once-consistent pace may now show anomalies, indicating the impending end of reproductive potential. It's not a goodbye so much as a shift, a transformation into a new stage of your womanhood.

The biochemical basis of perimenopause affects several different bodily systems in addition to the ovaries and hormones. Hormonal fluctuations cause small vibrations that are felt by the brain, bones, and cardiovascular system. In instance, estrogen contributes to heart health and bone density maintenance. Knowing these links gives you the ability to make decisions that are best for your general health.

Let's now discuss the brain, the complex command center that runs the entire operation. Hormonal changes during the perimenopause might affect mood and mental abilities. It is not unusual to go through periods of amnesia or emotional shifts. Consider it a part of the complex dance your brain does during this shift, an organic ebb and flow.

It's important to recognize that perimenopause is a unique experience in the middle of these changes. Because every woman's biological makeup is different, each woman's perimenopausal journey will have its own beat and song. The secret to getting through this stage with grace and understanding is to embrace your uniqueness.

A symphony of change, a harmonic interplay of hormones, organs, and systems, is the fundamental basis of perimenopause. It's a cooperative endeavor rather than a solitary performance that asks you to become acquainted with the complex functions of your body. Thus, let curiosity lead the way as you set out on your adventure, and allow the cordial murmurs of biology to reveal the splendor of the perimenopause.

Hormonal Changes and their Effects

Let's begin with the main performers, progesterone and estrogen. During the perimenopause, these two hormonal powerhouses take center stage, and their dance can have a profound effect on our bodies and thoughts.

The hormone known as "the queen of hormones," estrogen, begins to waltz to its own beat. Imagine that your estrogen levels suddenly drop. A number of changes may result from this, such as irregular menstrual periods and hot flashes that transport you to a tropical getaway. Furthermore, changes in estrogen can have an impact on the condition of our skeletons because it is essential for preserving bone density. It's as if estrogen were the conductor of a symphony, directing many facets of our health.

Let us not overlook progesterone, which serves as the auxiliary partner in this hormonal tango. Progesterone and estrogen frequently work well together. However, there may be difficult times in this connection during the perimenopause. Progesterone may fall short of estrogen, resulting in an imbalance that can induce mood swings and a hint of emotional instability.

The storyline surprise is that progesterone and estrogen are not the only factors at play. Other hormones that bring their own set of effects, such as cortisol and testosterone, join the party. Often connected to men, testosterone affects women's bodies in ways that affect desire and energy levels. Changes in testosterone levels during the perimenopause can impact our general energy and desire for intimacy.

And then there's our hormone of stress, cortisol. Stress can intensify the consequences of perimenopause, as if it weren't already an exciting time. Think of this pair of hormones as dance partners; one goes first, the other follows. Stress can cause cortisol to surge, which can affect our mood, weight, and even how well we sleep.

After getting to know the ensemble of players, let's examine how this hormonal drama affects our day-to-day existence. The most visible indicator is the irregular menstrual cycle, which is caused by the complex dance between progesterone and estrogen. At the most unexpected moments, hot flashes could show up as your unexpected guests and leave you feeling as though you've entered a sauna.

Mood swings are also important. Hormone fluctuations have the power to elevate even the most routine situations to exhilarating heights. You could be feeling extremely happy one minute and navigating through a sea of emotions the next. It's like a seesaw of hormones that constantly alerts us.

And there's the problem of sleep—or the absence of it. We may find ourselves tossing and turning in the early hours of the night due to hormonal fluctuations that disturb our sleep cycles. This can be the perfect storm for restless nights and foggy mornings, especially when combined with the stress element.

But don't worry, my dear reader. Regaining control over your body and mind starts with understanding these hormonal shifts. Even though it could be a rough journey, it can really help to approach this stage with humor and a little self-love. Thus, let's ride the hormone roller coaster with grace, resiliency, and a smile on our faces!

CHAPTER 2: Recognizing Perimenopausal Symptoms

Early Warning Signs

The perimenopause is a crucial stage that enters a woman's life subtly and frequently sneaks up on us unnoticed. Our everyday experiences are intertwined with a complex tapestry of change. Although there's no big reveal, there are early hints and soft prods from our bodies indicating the beginning of this life-changing experience.

Imagine yourself enjoying your morning coffee as you go through emails when all of a sudden you start to feel heated all over. A trace of sweat appears on your brow. They call them hot flashes. a condition that many women experience early in the perimenopause. It feels as though your body is gently tapping you on the shoulder to let you know that change is coming.

However, hot flashes are merely the prelude. You may also have fluctuations in your mood to go along with this pleasant feeling. You could be laughing so hard at a sitcom one minute and, during a commercial break, suddenly feeling like crying for no apparent reason. It seems as though your feelings have chosen to go on an exciting journey, discovering peaks and valleys you were unaware of.

Yes, but let's not overlook the erratic menstrual cycles, which are yet another subliminal indicator of impending change. It's possible that your monthly visitor, who was previously a dependable guest, is now hiding out on your calendar. In some months it shows up out of the blue, while in others it takes a long vacation, leaving you wondering if it's saying goodbye for forever.

Sleep disruptions are another uninvited guest that wants to stay. The quiet evenings you used to take for granted all of a sudden become a restless cacophony. Your nighttime companion may morph into insomnia, causing you to go through the day with heavy eyes and a strong desire for the illusive embrace of sound sleep.

Recognize the clear impact on your energy levels as you negotiate these early warning indicators. It's possible for fatigue to become a regular guest, making even the easiest chores seem difficult. It feels like your body is telling you to honor the rhythm of this developing journey, to slow down, and to accept periods of respite.

But do not be alarmed; these signals also herald times of resilience and self-discovery. You can discover an inner strength in the middle of the uncertainty that you were unaware of. Your capacity for flexibility and humor in the face of fluctuating hormones becomes evidence of the extraordinary spirit that characterizes womanhood.

In addition to the changes in the body and mind, there is a slight change in viewpoint. You might begin to doubt what society expects of you and welcome your newfound authenticity. Your internal compass takes center stage and becomes the leading force, directing you down a path paved with empowerment and self-acceptance as the cacophony of outside criticism subsides.

Thus, when you see these early warning indicators, consider them to be your body's gentle reminders to get to know yourself better rather than as disturbances. Accept the warmth of hot flashes, flow with the tides of your feelings, and go through the erratic cycles with curiosity.

Perimenopause is a special thread that weaves through the canvas of your experiences in the larger scheme of life. Every indication, every subtlety, is a brushstroke that adds to your story's masterwork. Thus, as you embark on this new chapter of your life, give a nod of cordial acknowledgment to the changes that lie ahead and approach it with an open mind and a spirit strong enough to welcome the dance of change.

Common Physical Symptoms

Our bodies go on an amazing adventure during the exhilarating roller coaster ride known as perimenopause, complete with a parade of physical symptoms that may cause us to snicker a little.

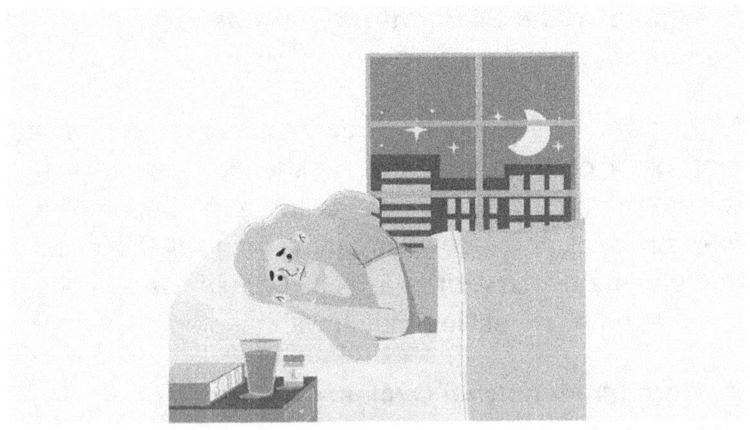

But don't worry—you're not going on this adventure alone. Let's explore the area of typical physical symptoms that occur during perimenopause, learning about the peculiarities and finding strategies to reduce the occasional hiccups.

1. Hot Flashes: The Uninvited Heatwave

Imagine being in the frozen food aisle of your neighborhood grocery store, but feeling like you're sunbathing in the Sahara with a sudden wave of heat.

Unquestionably the masters of perimenopausal physical theatrics, hot flashes can attack at any time, leaving you sweaty and confused. The favorable tidings? These sparks are fleeting, like an impromptu summertime shower of rain. Wear loose clothing, carry a portable fan, and have a little humor to stay cool.

2. Night Sweats: Midnight Adventures in Perspiration

Night sweats, the nighttime counterpart of hot flashes, may be a present from the perimenopause, as if that weren't enough. Fear not—breathable bedding and moisture-wicking sleepwear can be your reliable allies in this steamy bedtime drama. Your formerly serene sleep may become a wrestling match with tangled blankets.

3. Irregular Menstrual Cycles: The Dance of Unpredictability

Bid farewell to your old predictable menstrual cycle; perimenopause throws it a curveball. Expect irregular periods, shorter or longer cycles, and an unpredictable flow. It's like a dance party where the DJ is playing a remix of your favorite song – familiar, yet slightly offbeat. Keep track with a menstrual calendar and embrace the unpredictability with a sense of humor.

4. Sleep Disturbances: The Bedtime Balancing Act

Ahh, the elusive good night's sleep; the perimenopause may provide you with its cheeky antithesis. Sleepless evenings and insomnia may become frequent guests. To entice the Sandman back and bring peace back to your nights, set up a regular nighttime routine, cut back on caffeine, and establish a calm sleeping atmosphere.

5. Fatigue: The Unwelcome Visitor

Feel like you've run a marathon without leaving your living room? Fatigue during perimenopause can be like that sneaky neighbor who overstays their welcome. Prioritize rest, incorporate energizing foods into your diet, and consider light exercises to keep fatigue at bay.

6. Mood Swings: The Emotional Roller Coaster

Expect an emotional roller coaster because mood swings are a normal aspect of going through the perimenopause. You could be living life to the fullest one minute and wondering why you're not the same the next. Use self-compassion, mindfulness, and deep breathing techniques to take care of your mental health.

7. Weight Fluctuations: The Scale's Teasing Game

Weight gain, loss, or a mysterious combination of both can become your body's latest hobby during perimenopause. Instead of obsessing over the scale, focus on a balanced diet and regular exercise. Celebrate your body for all the incredible journeys it has taken you on.

8. Joint Pain: The Creaks and Groans

Ever have the impression that your joints are trying out for a drum group? Unexpectedly, perimenopause can bring on joint pain. Maintain your activity level with low-impact workouts, think about making nutritional adjustments, and speak with your healthcare professional for individualized advice.

9. Vaginal Dryness: The Intimate Drought

Intimacy might encounter a dry spell due to vaginal dryness. Fear not; lubricants and open communication with your partner can transform this challenge into an opportunity to strengthen your connection.

10. Memory Fog: The Forgetful Symphony

Put the memory fog to use if you start losing keys or forgetting why you entered a room. It's all part of the adventure to keep your mind sharp with brain workouts, eat a nutritious diet, and laugh at your occasional forgetfulness.

Your body is using the perimenopausal physical symptoms as a symphony, with each note playing a distinct melody that represents this transitional period. Accept your peculiarities, ask for help when you need it, and keep in mind that this is only the beginning of your incredible journey.

Emotional and Mental Changes

Emotional and mental changes are one of the most subtle and significant threads we come across in the complex tapestry of perimenopause. Imagine it as an emotional rollercoaster, a colorful mosaic of experiences that may make you laugh, cry, or just plain confused. But have no fear—understanding and accepting this emotional tornado is a vital first step in gracefully passing through this stage.

The hormonal orchestra in your body is always influencing your emotional landscape as it plays its intricate symphony. You can find yourself laughing so hard at a sitcom that you're on the edge of tears during a wonderful commercial. Emotions seem to be skating to a beat that only they can hear while donning their own pair of roller skates. The varying levels of progesterone and estrogen are the cause of this prevalent heightened emotional sensitivity.

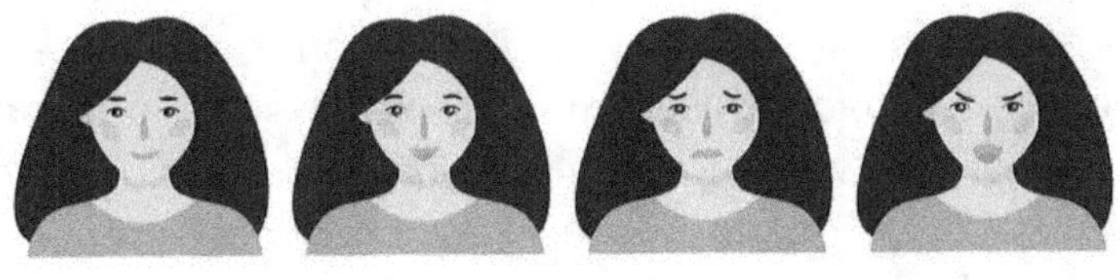

Conversely, there may be times when you feel as though your feelings are being muted. You can experience a brief loss of the vibrancy that once characterized your moods, leaving you with a muted emotional palette. It's important to understand that these changes are temporary, that the emotional rollercoaster has highs and lows, and that it's acceptable to occasionally glide slowly through periods of emotional peace.

During the perimenopause, anxiety and uneasiness may also manifest. Anxiety can take on a distinct form when it is combined with confusion about the changes that your body is going through and the expectations that society has for aging. It seems like you're standing on the brink of an exciting cliff, not knowing what's going to fall below. Here's where honest communication shines like a guiding light. Talk to dependable friends about your worries, or get advice from a medical expert who can provide you with peace of mind while you traverse this unfamiliar territory.

Depression may also make an appearance during the perimenopause. Hormonal fluctuations can have a negative impact on your mental health, so it's important to know the warning signals. Seeking professional help could be a good idea if you experience recurrent depressive symptoms or lose interest in past hobbies. Mental health is important and should be treated with the same care and attention as our physical health.

Developing resilience becomes essential to enduring these psychological and emotional shifts. Accept your own compassion for yourself and your own strength. Embrace a network of friends and family that are sympathetic and aware of the complexities involved in this journey. Take part in enjoyable activities and establish a mental haven where you can go when emotional storms threaten.

Recall that going through the perimenopause is a deep transition that affects every aspect of your life, not just a physical one. You give yourself the ability to get through this stage with a resilient and self-loving attitude by accepting and having faith in the emotional and mental shifts. Fasten your seatbelt, relish the journey, and let your feelings to surface—they are an essential component of the exquisite mosaic that defines your individuality.

CHAPTER 3: Navigating Hormonal Shifts

Estrogen Fluctuations

Greetings from the complex realm of estrogen, the hormone conductor that masterfully controls your body's ups and downs. You've probably come across the capricious dance of estrogen levels if you're perimenopausal. Don't worry—this amicable trip will reveal the secrets of estrogen swings and provide illuminating and empowering insights.

An Introduction to the Ballet of Estrogen

Think of your body as a well-tuned orchestra, with estrogen playing the lead role. This conductor becomes erratic and whimsical during perimenopause, resulting in what we lovingly refer to as "fluctuations." These variations signal the beginning of a new stage of life and are not a malfunction in the system but rather an inevitable aspect of growing older.

The Rise and Fall of Estrogen

Estrogen plays the lead role in the magnificent symphony of hormonal shifts, with a lovely crescendo and decrescendo. Estrogen levels can rise sharply in the early stages of perimenopause, like in an exciting musical finale. Your menstrual cycle may alter as a result of this surge, resulting in irregular periods that may catch you off guard.

On the other hand, as perimenopause advances, estrogen can choose to back off, resulting in quieter passages in the hormonal symphony. You may have symptoms including mood swings, heat flashes, and changes in the health of your vagina during these times. It's similar to the orchestra momentarily turning down the level so that certain instruments can have a more prominent role.

Balance in Hormonal Changes

Consider changes in estrogen levels as the organic progression of your body's hormonal harmony. The perimenopause journey has its highs and lows, just like any musical composition. Your experience may feel more harmonious if you realize that these variations are a typical aspect of the procedure.

How Menstrual Cycles Are Affected

Your menstrual cycle is controlled by estrogen, which also affects its rate and rhythm. You may notice variations in the length and intensity of your periods when estrogen levels alter. Certain cycles might conclude sooner, while others might unintentionally last longer. It's similar to the conductor experimenting with various tempos to produce a different piece every time.

Getting Around the Emotional Terrain

Not only is estrogen a hormone conductor, but it's also a major player in your life's emotional symphony. Changes in estrogen levels can have an impact on mood swings, giving you a sense of emotional rollercoaster. You could be engrossed in happy music one moment and a depressing melody the next.

To navigate perimenopause with grace, one must have a thorough understanding of these emotional nuances. You can develop emotional harmony by accepting the variety of your inner symphony, just as a trained musician adjusts to the shifting tones of a piece.

Choosing the Appropriate Tempo: Coping Techniques

As estrogen conducts the orchestra through its dynamic shifts, it's critical to arm yourself with self-management techniques. In times of elevated estrogen, doing stress-relieving exercises like yoga or meditation might provide a calming break from your regular schedule. In a similar vein, leading a healthy lifestyle can offer the required balance when estrogen levels are lower.

The Wisdom of Acceptance

The key in this gentle investigation of hormone changes is acceptance. By accepting the inherent cadence of your hormones, you can navigate the perimenopause with poise and self-awareness. Your journey through estrogen fluctuations has its own distinct charm, just like every musical composition does. It's a symphony of change that enriches and adds dimension to your life's tapestry.

Recall that you are not alone on this melodious trip through the ups and downs of perimenopause. Like a masterfully performed symphony, your body has the natural capacity to adjust and produce a stunning composition that is exclusively yours. Accept the ups and downs, find the positive in the shifts, and allow the amiable dance of estrogen lead you with assurance and style through this transforming phase.

Progesterone Variations

Progesterone is the main hormone during the perimenopause, part of the complex hormonal symphony that governs a woman's reproductive journey. Progesterone, which is sometimes called the "calming hormone," affects a woman's overall health as well as the menstrual cycle due to its cyclical fluctuations.

An Overview of the Progesterone Orchestra: An Understanding

Understanding progesterone's fundamental function is crucial to understanding the subtleties of its variants. In the second half of the menstrual cycle, the ovaries—more especially, the corpus luteum—produce the hormone progesterone. It plays a variety of roles, including influencing the lining of the uterus, controlling the menstrual cycle, and promoting early pregnancy.

Progesterone Throughout the Menstrual Cycle: The Monthly Dancing

Progesterone levels increase in the luteal phase of the menstrual cycle after ovulation. This surge creates a milieu that is conducive to a fertilized egg and primes the uterine lining for a possible pregnancy. Progesterone levels drop in the absence of fertilization, which initiates the menstrual cycle.

Variations in Perimenopausal Progesterone Levels

The progesterone tango takes on a new dimension during the perimenopausal journey. Menstrual cycle irregularities are caused by the ovaries' steady reduction in progesterone production as a woman approaches menopause. Hormone variations, such as a relative drop in progesterone relative to estrogen, are the hallmark of this phase.

Effect on Menstrual Cycles: The Random Pace

Menstrual cycle irregularity is one of the obvious impacts of progesterone changes during the perimenopause. Women may have irregular periods, shorter or longer cycles, or even miss menstruation entirely. The overall alterations in the landscape of reproduction are partly attributed to this erratic progesterone dance.

Mood Swings and Progesterone: Managing the Emotional Rollercoaster

Progesterone affects mood and emotional well-being significantly in addition to its involvement in reproduction. Perimenopause-related reductions in progesterone levels may be a factor in mood swings, impatience, and increased emotional sensitivity. Women are more equipped to negotiate the emotional terrain with resilience and self-awareness when they are aware of these variations.

Handling Symptoms: Techniques for Maintaining Progesterone Balance

Although the perimenopausal journey is accompanied by a normal reduction in progesterone, there are techniques to enhance hormonal equilibrium. Stress reduction, consistent exercise, and good nutrition are all very important in reducing the effects of progesterone fluctuations. During this stage, incorporating these lifestyle components might improve overall wellbeing.

Bone Health and Progesterone: An Essential Connection

Progesterone has an effect on bone health in addition to reproductive issues. Sustaining bone density requires adequate progesterone levels, and the reduction in progesterone during the perimenopause raises questions regarding the health of the bones. Women who are about to enter this period are urged to investigate food selections and lifestyle practices that promote bone density.

Examining Hormone Replacement Treatment (HRT): A Need for Balance

Hormone Replacement Therapy (HRT) may be an option for certain women whose progesterone fluctuations are causing severe symptoms. To treat symptoms, hormone replacement therapy (HRT) involves giving the body extra hormones, such as progesterone. But it's important to approach HRT cautiously, balancing the possible advantages against the hazards involved.

The Mind-Body Link: Holistic Methods for Endocrine Balance

When one acknowledges the complex relationship that exists between changes in hormones and mental health, holistic methods become critical. During periods of progesterone fluctuations, mind-body techniques like mindfulness, yoga, and meditation can be very helpful in reducing stress and fostering emotional balance.

Embracing the Journey: An Adaptive Tapestry

It is critical that women approach this life-changing journey with self-compassion and fortitude as they weave through the tapestry of progesterone fluctuations throughout perimenopause. Knowing the progesterone dance gives women insight into the changes they go through and gives them the ability to make decisions that will support their physical, emotional, and mental health.

In summary, changes in progesterone throughout the perimenopause are a normal aspect of the complex hormonal dance that characterizes a woman's reproductive cycle. Women can embrace the changing stages of life and set out on this path with confidence provided they comprehend and navigate these variances with knowledge.

Impact on Menstrual Cycles

The dynamic dance of menstruation, which is unique to each woman. Perimenopause invites us to a new beat as it taps us on the shoulder while we waltz through life. Let's talk about how this phase affects our formerly regular menstrual cycles.

First and foremost, visualize your monthly cycle as main instruments in a masterfully organized symphony, performed by hormones. Progesterone and estrogen alternately lead this complex dance, making sure everything goes together perfectly. The perimenopause, however, is like adding a jazz improvisation—it's full of character and a little erratic.

Your menstrual cycle irregularity is among the first obvious alterations. It sounds like the orchestra choosing to omit a beat or play a few more notes. If Aunt Flo begins fiddling with the schedule, decides to take a rain check, or shows up without warning, don't be shocked. This abnormality is frequently one of the first indications that the perimenopause is becoming more prominent.

Let's now discuss flow, specifically in relation to menstruation rather than art. Your menstrual cycle's length and volume may change during the perimenopause. A monthly visitor may prove to be too much for some, but a shorter, more brisk visit may be had by others. Your menstrual cycle seems to be experimenting with varied tempos, which keeps you alert.

Those well-known premenstrual companions, cravings and mood swings, may also be invited to the perimenopausal party. Hormonal changes have the power to escalate a mild chocolate craving into a full-blown cocoa addiction. And those changes in mood? Consider them emotional acrobatics: you may be laughing at a sitcom one minute and crying at a tearful commercial the next.

But have no fear, my friend; understanding is going to be your reliable dance partner on this voyage. Acknowledging these shifts gives you the confidence to take charge. Make a note of the tempo, rhythm, and any unexpected solos in your menstruation journal. It serves as your roadmap during this period of transition.

Accept self-care and navigate its ups and downs with the grace of an experienced dance partner. Make sure your diet is full of meals high in nutrients to help your body settle into its new routine. Drink plenty of water and exercise your body—whether it's a slow waltz or a fast salsa, do what feels good for you.

Seek out your tribe's assistance, open up about your experiences, and invite others to dance with you. The dance floor feels more welcoming when you have someone to laugh with about how unpredictable life can be or a shoulder to cry on during a particularly trying time.

To sum up, perimenopause is not the end of your menstrual dance, though it may give it some surprising twists. Think of it as a remix of the soundtrack of your life, where new and old songs collide. Accept the beat, swing with the modifications, and never forget that the dance goes on—beautifully, distinctively, and genuinely yours.

CHAPTER 4: Managing Physical Health

Nutritional Strategies

Your diet is a major factor in how your perimenopause unfolds, a colorful tapestry that shapes the trip. Embracing a cordial alliance with food is key to navigating this particular phase with grace and vigor; it's not just about what's on your plate.

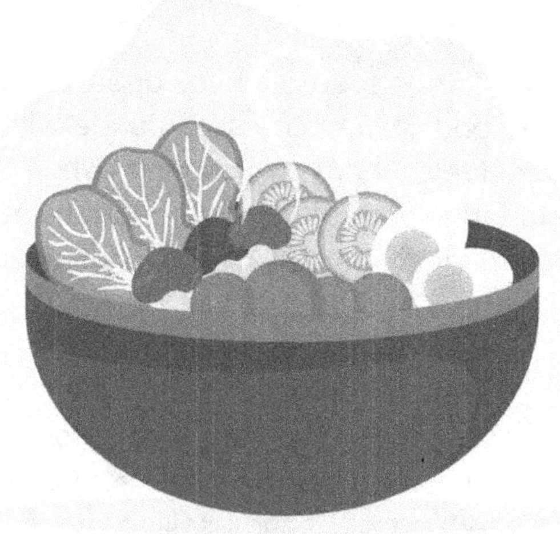

Let's start by discussing the two supernutrients: calcium and vitamin D. These energetic partners-in-crime are essential for preserving bone health, and during perimenopause, your bones will truly enjoy the affection. Trust me. To make sure your skeletal system is sturdy, make sure you consume plenty of dairy, leafy greens, and sunlight.

Let's now celebrate the effectiveness of omega-3 fatty acids. These hidden warriors provide a calming salve to the maelstrom of hormones. Walnuts, flaxseeds, and fatty fish all contain them. They are the backstage team, putting forth a lot of effort to control mood swings and inflammation.

The unsung hero of intestinal harmony is fiber. Fiber maintains the harmony of your digestive tract while hormones dance about you. Here, your best friends are fruits, veggies, and whole grains. They are a real win-win during periods of hormone fluctuation because they not only keep things going smoothly but also add to a feeling of fullness.

Not to be overlooked in the discussion of hormonal balance are phytoestrogens. These plant-based substances function as kind mediators between your hormones, brokering a peaceful agreement. They can be found in chickpeas, lentils, and soy products. They provide the body's mild reminder of estrogen, balancing everything out.

Your hidden weapon is staying hydrated. Water is a game-changer, not just an ordinary necessity. Sufficient hydration maintains your energy levels and aids in your body's adjustment to changes in hormones. Herbal teas, flavored water, and the occasional dash of real fruit juice will liven up your water game.

Finally, but no less importantly, savor antioxidants as though they were a guilt-free treat. Your antioxidant-rich companions are green tea, dark chocolate, and berries. They fight oxidative stress, promoting your general health and assisting your body in adapting to the changes with grace.

Recall that this is a helpful guide to support your body and spirit throughout perimenopause rather than a strict set of rules. Let the flavors, textures, and colors on your plate serve as a canvas to commemorate this wonderful journey you're on. Your body is a lifelong friend; cherish each mouthful of this nourishing journey and treat it with love.

Exercise and Fitness in Perimenopause

Welcome to the perimenopause, a stage of life when embracing fitness and exercise becomes a wonderful necessity rather than just a choice! Being active is crucial for promoting general well-being as our bodies go through this amazing transformation.

Understanding the Perimenopausal Landscape

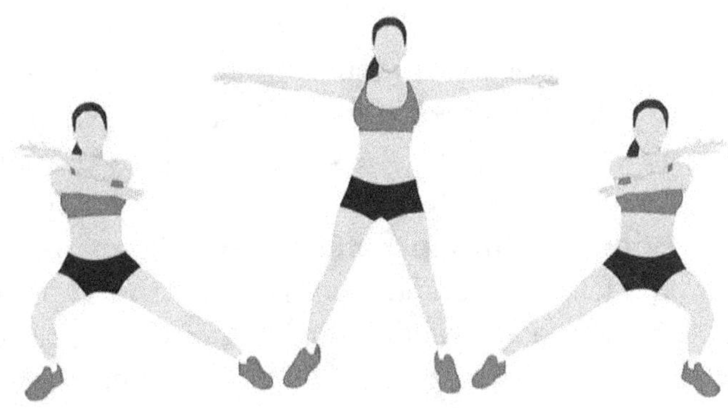

Visualize that when your body goes through hormonal gymnastics, exercise becomes a dependable partner in this dance of change. Hormonal changes, especially those related to progesterone and estrogen, can cause changes in muscle mass and metabolism during the perimenopause. Regular physical activity turns into an effective tool for gracefully navigating these transitions.

The Benefits of Exercise:

Let's talk about the incredible perks that exercise brings to the perimenopausal table:

1. **Mood Boosting Magic:** Exercise releases feel-good endorphins that can balance out the hormone roller coaster, making it a natural mood

enhancer. A more stable emotional state is what you'll be welcoming in place of mood swings.

2. **Metabolism Matters:** As our metabolism tends to slow down during perimenopause, maintaining a regular exercise routine can help counteract this natural process. It's not just about fitting into your favorite jeans – it's about keeping your body running smoothly.

3. **Bone Health Support:** Bone density can also be impacted by perimenopausal hormonal changes. Walking and strength training are two examples of weight-bearing activities that can help you maintain bone health and lower your risk of osteoporosis.

4. **Sleeping Beauty Mode:** Quality sleep can become elusive during perimenopause, but fear not – exercise can come to the rescue. Regular physical activity helps regulate sleep patterns, ensuring you wake up feeling refreshed and ready to tackle the day.

Finding Your Exercise Groove:

The secret to a fruitful perimenopausal fitness journey is to engage in activities you truly love. It's about adding activity into your daily life in a way that makes you feel good, not about following a strict regimen.

1. **Mix it Up:** Examine a range of workouts, such as strength training, swimming, and brisk walks and yoga. Changing up your regimen guarantees a

well-rounded approach to training in addition to keeping things interesting.

2. **Listen to Your Body:** Your body is a wise guide. Pay attention to how it responds to different types of exercise. If something doesn't feel right, modify or switch it up. The goal is to feel energized, not depleted.

3. **Make it Social:** Take a lesson, get a friend, or just dance in your home room. Including others in exercise not only adds enjoyment but also offers a network of support during this time of transition.

Recall that accepting growth is the goal here, not reaching perfection. Find something that moves you, both literally and figuratively. It may be a yoga class, a dance party in your living room, or a stroll in the morning. Welcome to a new chapter in which working out is a celebration of your strong, resilient self rather than merely a routine. Let's go on our journey!

Sleep Hygiene and Its Importance

Sleep is frequently neglected in the rush of daily life in favor of obligations, deadlines, and the plethora of activities that keep us moving all the time. However, the value of getting a good night's sleep cannot be emphasized. Let me introduce you to the world of sleep hygiene, a series of habits that help you have restful nights and refreshed days.

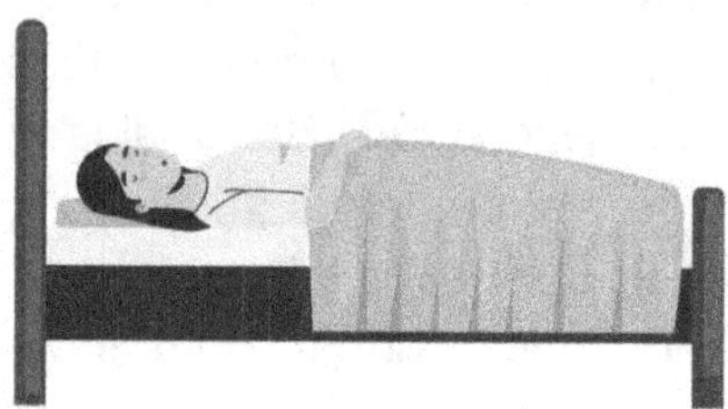

Understanding Sleep Hygiene:

While cleaning your bedroom's flooring and doing your laundry are good things to do, they are not the main components of good sleep hygiene! Rather, it's a set of routines and behaviors that establish the perfect environment for restful sleep. Consider it a recipe for calm that lets your body and mind relax.

The Bedtime Ritual:

Think of your nightly ritual as a smooth transition from the stresses of the day to the peace and quiet of the night. Take part in activities that let your body know when it's time to relax. Find a method that works for you, whether it's reading a book, having a warm bath, or using relaxation techniques.

Create a Sleep Sanctuary: Your bedroom ought to be a peaceful haven. Maintain it calm, dark, and cold. Invest in a mattress that offers the support your body requires and cozy bedding. Electronic devices that cause your body to produce blue light and interfere with your sleep-wake cycle should be banned.

Consistent Sleep Schedule:

Routine is cherished by our bodies, and the way you sleep is no different. Even on the weekends, try to maintain a regular wake-up and bedtime schedule. This facilitates natural sleep and wakefulness by balancing your body's internal schedule.

Mind Your Meals and Beverages:

Your sleep is directly impacted by the food you eat. Heavy meals should be avoided right before bed because they can be uncomfortable. Caffeine and nicotine are stimulants that might make it difficult for you to fall asleep and stay asleep.

Get Moving During the Day:

Regular physical activity is a natural sleep aid. However, try to finish your workout a few hours before bedtime to allow your body temperature to drop, signaling that it's time to wind down.

Tech Timeout:

The blue light that screens create can interfere with your sleep, even while going through your phone or binge-watching your favorite show can seem like a soothing way to finish the day. Try to turn off electronics at least one hour before going to bed.

The Power of Naps:

Short naps can be rejuvenating, but avoid lengthy siestas, especially in the late afternoon. This could interfere with your ability to fall asleep at night.

Managing Stress:

A cluttered mind can keep you tossing and turning. Practice stress-reducing techniques, such as meditation or deep-breathing exercises, to calm your mind before bedtime.

Seek Professional Help When Needed:

A healthcare professional's knowledge may be necessary if persistent sleep problems persist. Don't be afraid to ask for help if, despite practicing excellent sleep hygiene, you are still having trouble getting enough sleep.

Essentially, practicing good sleep hygiene is your ticket to a restful, deep sleep. You may create an environment where sleep is valued as an ally on your path to general well-being by adopting these easy yet powerful habits into your daily routine. Those who practice good sleep hygiene can look forward to sweet dreams!

CHAPTER 5: Emotional Well-being During Perimenopause

Addressing Mood Swings

The emotional rollercoaster that is perimenopause! Contrary to popular belief, mood fluctuations are not unique to you. Imagine it as a distinct song of midlife, with each note contributing to the overall symphony of hormonal shifts.

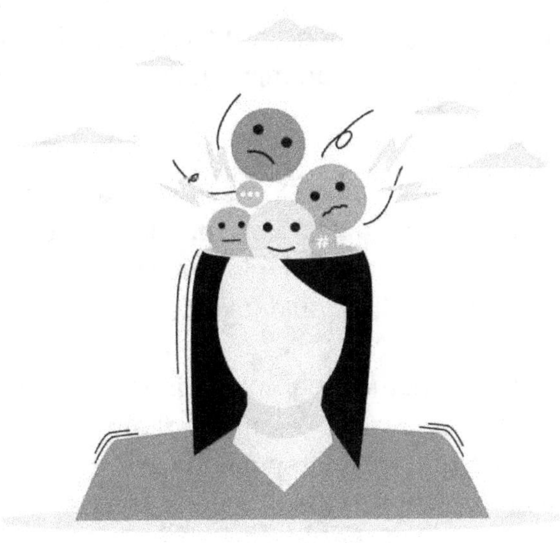

First and foremost, it's critical to understand that mood swings are a normal aspect of the perimenopausal experience. Hormones, those sneaky little messengers, like to hide and seek, giving you sudden bursts of happiness or frustration—or perhaps a little bit of both.

It's important to know the rhythm of your body. Breathe deeply when those mood swings happen. Hold on. Think back. You're managing a transition that's as unique as you are; you're not losing your marbles. Accept the ups and downs of life with a hint of self-compassion.

Your ally is communication. Tell your family and friends the secret. Tell them you're riding the hormonal wave, and it may feel like a storm at times. They'll be grateful for the heads-up, and I promise that being honest about it can strengthen your bond.

Self-care turns into your closest ally. Treat yourself to joyful pursuits, like a leisurely stroll, a nice book, or some time spent with your closest friends and family. Your emotional health should take center stage.

Think about implementing mindfulness exercises into your everyday schedule. Yoga, meditation, or even just a short period of calm introspection can be very effective strategies for traversing the emotional terrain.

And never forget that asking for help from an expert is a strength, not a weakness. If mood fluctuations become too much to handle or are ongoing, talking with a healthcare professional can be very insightful and supportive.

Essentially, managing mood swings during perimenopause involves accepting the journey, adjusting with a dash of humor, and acknowledging that, similar to a well-written novel, your story is becoming increasingly intricate.

Coping with Anxiety and Depression

During life's ups and downs, a lot of us struggle with the unwanted company of despair and anxiety. It's similar to navigating choppy waters, but let's take a minute to discuss how to ride those waves with compassion and resiliency.

First and foremost, realize that this experience is not unique to you. Recognizing that anxiety and sadness are normal human emotions is the first step toward recovery. It's consoling to know you're not alone on the rollercoaster, especially when everything else seems chaotic.

If you find that these feelings are too much to handle, you might want to ask for help from people in your immediate vicinity. Talk to your loved ones about how you're feeling; let them be your compass through choppy waters. Sometimes there's a huge release from just putting your ideas into words.

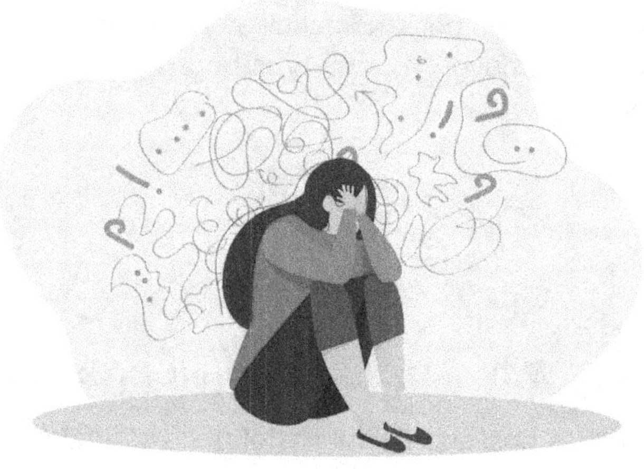

You can also use mindfulness as an anchor during a storm. Accept the current moment, let go of the past, and fight the impulse to think about the future, which is unknown. By practicing mindfulness, you can help lessen the hold that anxiety and despair have over you.

Establishing a routine can offer stability and organization. Achievable but modest objectives may save your life. Appreciate the small wins since they serve as stepping stones for bigger ones. The goal is to instill a feeling of purpose daily.

Engaging in physical activity can be a powerful remedy for emotional instability. Take part in enjoyable activities that will make you move. The endorphins that are created after an intense workout or a leisurely walk in the outdoors can act as a potent counterbalance to the negative effects of anxiety and sadness.

Think about the fuel you are giving your body. A balanced diet can be a helpful ally in maintaining mental health, as nutrition plays a critical role in mental health. Drink plenty of water, eat healthfully, and take time to enjoy every bite—a comprehensive strategy that nourishes your body and mind.

Mind-body techniques, like yoga and meditation, have the potential to change lives. These age-old forms of expression provide a haven for introspection and introspection. They want to embrace reality with a fresh sense of clarity and tranquility rather than run away from it.

Knowing when to seek expert assistance is essential. Counselors and therapists are qualified to help you navigate these emotional waters. Seeking them advice is a brave step toward understanding and taking control of your mental health, not a show of weakness.

And lastly, practice self-compassion. The process of healing is not a straight line; rather, it is an oscillation. Accept the highs and lows, realizing that every experience is a chapter in your own story.

Remind yourself that you are stronger than you realize when managing your anxiety and sadness. Like a strong sailor navigating a storm, you have the inner power to overcome the obstacles in life. It is possible to get out of the shadows and into the sunlight of a happier, more fulfilled existence with the help of others, self-compassion, and proactive actions.

Building Resilience

During the ups and downs of perimenopause, developing resilience becomes an effective strategy for getting through this life-changing stage. Resilience can be thought of as your loyal friend who gives you the fortitude to endure the hormonal storms and come out stronger on the other side.

First and foremost, it's critical to understand that resilience is about accepting obstacles with a growth-oriented perspective rather than dismissing them. Recognize the mental and physical changes your body is going through. You establish resilience by being aware of and tolerant of these changes.

Make sure you have a strong support system around you. Talk about your experiences with loved ones, friends, and support groups. Resilience is fostered by connection; realizing you're not traveling alone gives you a sense of community that helps you get through difficult times. Having candid discussions also helps to dispel the stigma associated with perimenopause, promoting empathy and understanding.

Accept your own compassion. Show yourself the same compassion and consideration that you so freely extend to others. Unexpected difficulties are a common part of perimenopause, and it's acceptable to not know everything. Give yourself the room you need to develop, learn, and adjust without the burden of irrational expectations.

Develop wholesome routines that feed your body and mind. Frequent exercise has a dramatic impact on mental resilience in addition to improving physical well-being. Find things that make you happy and relieve tension, whether it's yoga, dancing, or taking a quick stroll.

Both mindfulness and relaxation methods have their advantages. Include techniques like mindfulness, meditation, and deep breathing in your everyday routine. These not only aid in stress management but also improve your capacity to overcome difficult situations.

Set attainable objectives and acknowledge minor successes. Since resilience is fueled by a sense of achievement, breaking down more difficult activities into smaller ones enables you to go forward steadily. Honor your victories, no matter how tiny, and use them as a springboard to conquer bigger obstacles.

Lastly, keep an optimistic mindset. Give up on things you cannot control and concentrate on what you can. Having a resilient attitude entails seeing every problem as a chance for personal development and adjusting to change with optimism.

During the perimenopause, developing resilience is a lifelong process that involves constant self-reflection and adjustment. Through cultivating a resilient mindset and implementing these techniques on a daily basis, you prepare yourself to face perimenopause with grace, fortitude, and an upbeat spirit, ready to face any challenge that may arise.

CHAPTER 6: Relationships and Communication

Effect of Hormonal Changes on Relationships

Hormonal fluctuations during perimenopause are typically crucial in determining the dynamics of relationships in the complex dance of life. Women's emotional landscapes change in tandem with the fluctuations of hormones like progesterone and estrogen, which can have an impact on relationships with friends, family, and lovers.

The unpredictable nature of this hormonal journey is one of its main features. Hormonal changes can cause an emotional rollercoaster that is difficult for the person experiencing them as well as those around them. When partners see their loved ones struggle with mood swings, impatience, and heightened emotions, they may find themselves in unfamiliar territory.

During this stage, communication becomes crucial. Understanding and empathy are built on the foundation of candid and open communication. It's critical for partners to understand that these changes are a reflection of internal biological changes rather than personal assaults. A supportive atmosphere can be created by just acknowledging these hormonal changes.

Empathy turns into a potent instrument for preserving harmony in relationships. Partners who make an effort to comprehend the subtle emotional changes associated with perimenopause show a high degree of support. Being a consoling presence, ready to change with the times, and a listening ear become priceless assets.

Furthermore, it's critical to keep in mind that these hormone shifts affect more people than just the individual going through them. They set off a chain reaction that affects everyone inside their emotional sphere. It may also be necessary for friends and family to modify their expectations and reactions, encouraging a team effort to overcome the difficulties brought on by perimenopausal hormone changes.

Hormonal fluctuations have an impact on the level of intimacy as well. Some women could feel less lustful, but others might become more aware of their sensuality. In order to create a secure space in which to explore this area of their relationship, partners must be open in communicating about their wants, anxieties, and desires.

It also takes some flexibility to ride these hormonal waves. It could be necessary to modify what previously worked, and partners would have to become used to new routines and coping techniques. This flexibility makes the relationship more resilient and helps it weather any storms that may arise from hormonal fluctuations.

The demand for shared responsibility changes as partnerships do. By actively participating in the creation of a supportive atmosphere, partners can help the individual going through perimenopause efficiently manage their energy levels by splitting up domestic responsibilities. This cooperative method strengthens the idea that adjusting to hormonal changes is a shared journey and promotes a sense of teamwork.

No matter how minor the victory, it becomes imperative to celebrate it. Rewarding perseverance and strength in the face of adversity strengthens a couple's relationship. It's a time to give thanks for the silent times of understanding, the laughs shared, and the steadfast support that gets you through the ups and downs of hormones.

In summary, the impact of hormone fluctuations on romantic relationships during the perimenopause is a complex process. It calls for endurance, comprehension, and a dedication to progress. In addition to fortifying their bond, partners who skillfully negotiate this challenging terrain with empathy, candor, and flexibility also enhance the general well being of the individual going through these hormonal changes. Accepting the rhythm of change in life's dance becomes a harmonious, shared experience.

Communicating with Partners, Family, and Friends

Open communication with your loved ones—your partners, family, and friends—is one of the most important tasks. Together, we can fortify ties and establish a network of support as we navigate this period of transition, which will facilitate an easier journey for all parties.

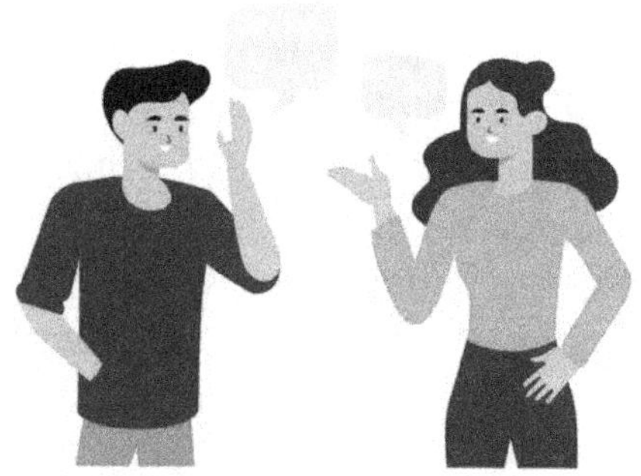

Consider the shifting threads of your perimenopausal feelings as a vibrant tapestry. With your spouse, sharing this tapestry may be an empowering and vulnerable experience. First, choose a quiet time to speak that is free from interruptions. Tell them how you're feeling, describe the experiences you're having, and ask them to help you make sense of this new phase of your life.

Family is essential in providing a solid support system during the perimenopause. It's important to keep in mind that your family is going through changes as well, even while you may be going through physical and mental changes. Open communication helps everyone understand the distinct difficulties that each member encounters by acting as a bridge that links the dots.

The strands of friendship are what give the fabric of life its color. Talking to others about your experiences throughout perimenopause can be reassuring and comforting. If you approach these discussions with genuineness, you might discover that your friends have gone through similar things or have insightful things to say. A sincere chat or a good chuckle might create an understanding that is not expressed.

Empathy is essential to good communication. Even though your partner might not fully understand the perimenopause, they can still be a helpful companion if you have patience and share experiences with each other. Urge them to participate in activities that enhance general well-being, go to doctor's appointments together, and ask questions.

Open communication can improve family relations and lead to more harmony. Family members can be adjusting to changes in routines and emotions while you deal with your own hormone variations. While you listen to their viewpoint, share your own as well. To improve the bonds between family members, identify a common ground and acknowledge the adjustments that everyone is making.

There is a special kind of friendship among those that can withstand change's storms. Talk honestly about your experiences, but listen to what they have to say as well. Through these talks, you could find that you can laugh together through difficult times or that you can pick up coping skills from one another. When you allow vulnerability to be a two-way street, friendships become a source of unwavering support.

No matter how tiny the victory may be, it's important to recognize it and appreciate the efforts your loved ones, friends, and partners have made to comprehend and encourage you. Thank them for their kindness, endurance, and willingness to travel with you on this adventure.

Recall that communication is an ongoing process. It's a continuous conversation that changes as you go through the perimenopause. Share your feelings with your loved ones and encourage them to share theirs by checking in with them on a frequent basis. Everyone takes an active part in the shared story of this transforming era as a result of this reciprocal exchange, which strengthens the sense of togetherness among people.

The communication threads weave a story of mutual support, understanding, and connection in the larger scheme of life. When you approach these talks with an open mind, you'll discover that friends, family, and partners can be your most powerful allies as you navigate the perimenopause dance.

Nurturing Intimacy in Midlife

Fostering connection with our partners becomes an art as we elegantly navigate this chapter of our lives; it calls for consideration, understanding, and a hint of spontaneity.

Numerous changes, both emotional and physical, are frequently associated with midlife. Maintaining and growing closeness can feel like a delicate balancing act during these changes. However, it's also the moment when our relationships with our partners have the potential to deepen and become more complex.

The foundation of any successful relationship is communication, thus this is an important factor. The middle years provide an opportunity to have deep talks about the complexities of our goals, anxieties, and wants. It's about exposing our innermost thoughts and feelings and accepting vulnerability. Whether it's a peaceful evening on the porch or an impromptu weekend trip, making time for candid conversation builds the emotional closeness that keeps partnerships strong.

Another essential component is being aware of each other's evolving demands. Changes in libido, energy levels, and even thoughts on relationships are frequently brought about by midlife. An even more fulfilling and harmonious relationship might result from taking the time to jointly investigate and understand these changes. The ability to adjust, show empathy, and have patience are the qualities that can turn obstacles into chances for development.

Playfulness is necessary to discover new aspects of closeness. Midlife ought to be a period of emancipation rather than restriction. A relationship gets excited when partners rediscover the joy of laughing together, attempt new things, or rekindle long-forgotten passions. This lively relationship breathes new life into it and supports the notion that intimacy is a journey that is always changing.

In midlife, physical intimacy also becomes more important. Fostering a deeper connection means accepting and lovingly embracing the changes our bodies go through. Discovering new ways to connect and enjoy each other via exploration and shared adventure is how sensuality transforms into a shared adventure. Rewriting the story of physical intimacy and appreciating the beauty of bodies that have endured time spent together is the goal.

In midlife, spontaneity becomes a valued ally in fostering relationships. Relationships are enhanced by spontaneous acts of love, such as surprising your lover with a passionate note, organizing an unplanned date night, or just showing affection when it's not expected. They act as a constant reminder that love is not constrained by regularity and instead flourishes in the unforeseen and unplanned.

Midlife offers a chance to plan for the future and to share dreams with others. Couples find themselves with more time to pursue shared passions and goals as children leave the nest and careers either reach new heights or shift. Developing a shared vision for the future—whether it involves vacation destinations, artistic endeavors, or volunteer work—adds a level of purpose that fosters intimacy.

In the vast scheme of midlife, fostering closeness is a joy rather than a chore. It's a recognition of the path taken together and a look forward to future adventures. It's about building a mosaic of shared experiences, love, and connection that only gets stronger with time—embracing life's ups and downs with your spouse by your side. So let the flames of intimacy burn strong, illuminating this lovely stage of life with a loving glow.

Stress Management Techniques

When women enter the perimenopausal stage, stress management becomes essential to preserving general health. A distinct set of difficulties may arise during this time due to hormonal changes and life transitions. Thankfully, there are a number of stress-reduction strategies that can enable women to move through this stage with resilience and ease.

Mindfulness meditation is one useful tactic. Stress levels can be considerably lowered by setting aside a little amount of time each day to sit still, concentrate on the breath, and raise awareness of the present moment. In addition to promoting mental calmness, mindfulness enables women to develop a closer bond with their bodies and an inner sense of tranquility.

Regular exercise is another effective strategy for reducing stress. Endorphins are the body's natural mood enhancers, and exercise has been shown to release them, which can reduce stress and lift your spirits. A lasting stress management technique starts with selecting an activity that fits into one's lifestyle and gives delight, whether that activity be strength training, yoga, or a brisk walk.

During the perimenopause, social support networks can be quite beneficial in reducing stress. Talking to friends, family, or support groups about struggles, victories, and experiences can make one feel less alone and validated. In addition to enhancing emotional health, strong social ties serve as a constant reminder that women are not experiencing perimenopause alone.

Making self-care a priority is essential. Taking time for oneself is not a luxury, but a need in the midst of all the duties and changes. This might be anything from curling up with a favorite hobby to reading a book or having a nice bath. Women who set aside time for self-care practices can refuel and handle the rigors of everyday life more effectively.

During the perimenopause, maintaining a nutritious diet is crucial for stress management. Eating foods high in nutrients, like fruits, vegetables, healthy grains, and lean meats, can improve emotional and physical health. Reducing intake of processed foods, refined carbohydrates, and caffeine can help control energy levels and encourage a more stable emotional state.

One of the most important stress-reduction techniques is learning to set reasonable expectations. Many life transitions, such as changes in family interactions and job paths, frequently occur around the time of perimenopause. One way to release tension and lessen pressure is to realize that you can't accomplish everything flawlessly and acknowledge that. The perimenopause can be easier to navigate if reasonable goals are set and duties are divided into small, doable increments.

Getting enough sleep is essential for managing stress and maintaining general health. Stress levels can rise as a result of sleep patterns being disturbed by hormonal shifts during the perimenopause. Better sleep quality can be achieved by establishing a regular bedtime pattern, making a calm sleeping environment, and avoiding stimulants just before bed.

Getting professional help, like therapy or counseling, can be very helpful for some women in controlling their stress levels. A qualified therapist can offer strategies for overcoming the psychological difficulties associated with perimenopause, as well as individualized support and assistance.

In summary, perimenopausal stress management calls for a comprehensive strategy that takes into account social, emotional, and physical health. Women can traverse the perimenopausal journey with resilience, grace, and a sense of empowerment by embracing mindfulness, regular exercise, social connections, self-care routines, a nutritious diet, realistic expectations, quality sleep, and professional support.

Career and Life Planning

As women negotiate this transitional era, career and life planning take center stage in the dynamic terrain of the perimenopause. This is the moment when setting new priorities and coordinating one's personal and professional objectives becomes not only necessary but also relevant.

Women frequently consider their employment paths when their hormones fluctuate. Now is the perfect time to assess if the current course still aligns with their goals. Accepting change becomes a mantra, and realizing that the perimenopausal experience can mark the beginning of an exciting new chapter full of opportunities is empowering.

Recalibrating goals is one way that career transitions can take shape; they don't always require a drastic change in direction. Maybe it's time to concentrate on passion projects or look into professional development opportunities. During this stage, networking becomes a useful tool for connecting with peers or mentors who have experienced similar transitions and building a supportive group.

Life planning is not just for work; it also includes relationships, general well-being, and personal goals. It entails examining inwardly what gives happiness and contentment. Perhaps now is the ideal time to take that long-awaited vacation, pick up a new skill, or strengthen bonds with loved ones.

During the perimenopause, juggling a professional and personal life requires admitting when self-care is necessary. This can be as easy as creating a daily schedule that supports both physical and emotional well-being. The maintenance of general well-being is critically dependent on regular exercise, mindfulness training, and restful sleep.

During this stage, adaptability becomes a crucial ally. Accept the fluidity of perimenopause and see it as a chance to mold a life and profession that are more in line with your own goals and ideals. Not only is this a time of change, but it's also a time of empowerment and self-discovery, with each choice you make pointing you in the direction of a more genuine and satisfying future.

Creating a Supportive Environment

During perimenopause, creating a supportive environment is like creating a warm embrace that surrounds you during a life-changing stage. It becomes vital to surround yourself with supportive surroundings as you negotiate the ups and downs of hormonal shifts. This is a mild look at creating an atmosphere that supports resilience and well-being.

Understanding Emotional Needs:

First of all, accept the emotional terrain that perimenopause presents. A wide range of emotions, including happiness, uncertainty, nostalgia, and even vulnerable moments, are associated with this time. It's important to communicate openly because people close to you might not understand all the subtleties of this trip. Communicate your wants, share your experiences, and open up to your loved ones about how you're feeling.

Creating Open Dialogues:

Building a supportive environment involves fostering open dialogues with your closest circles. Encourage conversations about perimenopause; dispel myths and share reliable information. This not only demystifies the process but also helps those around you understand the shifts you're going through. A family or friend who comprehends the journey is better equipped to offer the support you need.

Flexibility and Understanding:

Flexibility throughout hormonal changes is a valuable quality. Accept that your choices and needs may change. Whether it's some alone time, a listening ear, or a small act of kindness, be clear about what supports you. With this knowledge, those around you can adjust to your changing needs and create a setting that moves with the beat of your adventure.

Practical Support:

Help with practical matters can be just as important as emotional support. Stress can be reduced by doing small things like helping with daily chores or splitting household duties. A supportive atmosphere is one in which people who are close to you voluntarily take on more responsibility as necessary. This relieves the physical strain while also reaffirming that you're not going through perimenopause by yourself.

Empathy and Patience:

A supportive environment thrives on empathy and patience. Understand that the symptoms of perimenopause vary widely, and there's no one-size-fits-all solution. Patience becomes a balm, soothing the rough edges of emotional turbulence. When those around you approach the journey with empathy, it creates a safe haven where you feel understood and accepted.

Encouraging Self-Care:

One of the most important aspects of perimenopause navigation is self-care. Your self-care practices are celebrated and encouraged in a caring setting. Making time for hobbies, nature walks, or quiet times with a book should be your top priorities when it comes to activities that lift your soul. When people you care about actively support your efforts at self-care, it serves as a reminder of how important it is to take care of yourself during this critical stage.

All it takes to create a friendly environment for perimenopausal women is to weave a tapestry of compassion, understanding, and helpful advice. It's about building relationships that support one another through times of transition. By creating an atmosphere like this, you contribute to a culture of compassion and support that goes far beyond your own journey in addition to improving your own well-being.

CHAPTER 8: Hormone Replacement Therapy (HRT) Explained

Overview of Hormone Replacement Therapy

The dance of the hormones, a symphony that plays out the complex balance of our health. Women move through life's stages with elegance, but eventually the beat shifts and the focus shifts to the perimenopause. It's a state of flux, a time when our bodies experience major hormonal changes that bring about a wide range of mental and physical changes. Hormone Replacement Therapy (HRT) is a common source of comfort and support for many women on this ever changing path.

A Quick Introduction to Hormone Replacement Therapy

Imagine a busy stage where progesterone and estrogen used to be the main performers, flawlessly preserving reproductive health. But as the story goes on, during perimenopause, these hormones start to take a bow, creating a hole that can be filled by HRT as an encore.

Act I: Setting the Scene - What is Hormone Replacement Therapy?

Hormone Replacement Therapy (HRT) is a medical intervention that is used to supplement a woman's body during the perimenopause and menopause to replace the diminishing levels of estrogen and, occasionally, progesterone. Its main objective? to relieve the very difficult symptoms that come with this inevitable change in life.

Act II: Participants - Different Kinds of Hormone Replacement Therapy

Here come the characters: many HRT incarnations, each with its own script. There are two primary kinds: combination hormone therapy (CHT), which contains both progestin and estrogen for women with an intact uterus, and estrogen-only therapy (ET) for women who have had hysterectomy.

As the main character, estrogen captivates the audience by relieving vaginal dryness, nocturnal sweats, and hot flashes. The helpful co-star, progestin, is essential for uterine lining protection.

Act III: Hormone Replacement Therapy's Advantages Thickens the Plot

The advantages of HRT are now in the forefront as the curtain rises. This treatment turns into a lifesaver for a lot of ladies, providing a break from the chaotic world of perimenopausal symptoms. The emotional upheaval subsides, sleep disturbances settle in, and hot flashes fade into the background.

However, the story goes beyond only treating symptoms; HRT also helps to stop bone loss, which lowers the chance of osteoporosis and fractures. It might also improve heart health by influencing cholesterol levels and thereby lowering the risk of cardiovascular illnesses.

Act IV: The Critics: Risks and Controversies

But critics are inevitable with any great show, and HRT is no exception. Many have expressed worries about the script's possible hazards and adverse effects after it was carefully examined. The cast struggles with talking about how using some types of HRT increases the risk of blood clots, strokes, and breast cancer. Deciding to use HRT requires careful thought and discussion with medical professionals because it's a complex balancing act between the risks and benefits.

Act V: The Individual Path - Tailored Methods of Hormone Replacement Therapy

This story is beautiful because it is unique. Women react differently to hormone replacement therapy, just as no two experience perimenopause in the same way. While some could experience significant relief, others might look for other options. The secret is to recognize that every woman's narrative is different and to adjust hormone replacement therapy accordingly.

Act VI: The Backstage - Hormone Replacement Therapy Monitoring and Adjustments

Healthcare professionals act as vital directors behind the scenes, keeping an eye on the performance and modifying the dosage as necessary. Frequent check-ins guarantee that the balance between potential dangers and symptom treatment stays in place.

Act VII: The Options - Examining Different Routes

It's critical to understand that HRT is only one play in the vast drama of perimenopausal management as the last act draws near. Some women might decide to look into complementary and alternative therapy, like mind-body techniques, herbal supplements, or lifestyle modifications. The decision is quite personal, and the story can be changed to reflect personal tastes and ideals.

Act VIII: Accepting the Next Chapter - The Grand Finale

HRT might not be the perfect solution for every woman as the perimenopausal stage draws to a close. Some say goodbye to the limelight and welcome the next phase of their lives without the use of hormone supplements. At the grand finale, women are resilient and empowered, confidently navigating the unfamiliar region of menopause.

Epilogue: A Personal Choice

HRT becomes a crucial character in this dynamic play, providing comfort and assistance to individuals facing the difficulties of perimenopause. It's a personal decision shaped by personal histories, personal ideals, and health-related factors. The story may play out differently for every woman, but the general idea is always the same: going through the perimenopause is a life-changing experience, and hormone replacement therapy is only one instrument in a variety of tools that can help women navigate this incredible trip

Pros and Cons

Making the choice to investigate Hormone Replacement Therapy (HRT) in the perimenopause is like choosing a route that has both bright spots and shady areas. It's critical to realize that choosing HRT is a very personal decision that needs careful deliberation. Let's take a closer look at the advantages and disadvantages of hormone replacement therapy.

Pros:

1. Symptom Alleviation: HRT frequently proves to be a lifesaver, successfully relieving the uncomfortable symptoms associated with the perimenopause. Hormonal replacement therapy can provide a more tranquil passage through the turbulent waters of this transitional stage, reducing hot flashes and mood swings.

2. Better Quality of Life: Many women discover that using HRT improves their general well-being. Reduction of symptoms not only improves daily quality of life but also cultivates optimism, allowing for a more complete enjoyment of life's pleasures.

3. Support for Bone Health: Hormones are essential for preserving bone density. By lowering the risk of osteoporosis and fractures, HRT can help improve bone health and provide a strong basis for an active lifestyle.

4. Heart Health: Research points to the possibility that hormone replacement therapy (HRT) may improve cholesterol and lower the risk of heart disease. This feature adds a cardiovascular cherry on top of the hormonal storm cloud.

5. Cognitive Benefits: Research suggests a connection between HRT and cognitive performance. Hormone replacement therapy is thought to have a preventive impact against cognitive decline, which is a big plus for those who are worried about their mental health.

Cons:

1. Increased Health problems: The main issue surrounding HRT is the possible rise in a number of health problems. These might include a higher chance of stroke, blood clots, and breast cancer. It's critical that anyone thinking about HRT have a detailed discussion about these dangers with their healthcare physician.

2. Individual Variances: There are differences amongst HRT treatments. What fits one lady perfectly may not work the same way for another. One significant drawback of hormonal replacement therapy is the wide range of individual reactions, which emphasizes the need for individualized medical advice.

3. adverse Effects: HRT may have a variety of adverse effects, just like any medical procedure. Breast discomfort and headaches are a few examples of them. Even though these adverse impacts aren't always present, they should be taken into account while making decisions.

4. Timing Is Important: When starting hormone replacement therapy (HRT), there are potential effects and hazards. Delaying the onset of hormone replacement therapy (HRT) during the postmenopausal phase may increase the risk of some health problems, so it's important to carefully consider whether it's best for each individual.

5. Vigilant Monitoring Is Needed: Adhering to HRT Calls for Vigilant Monitoring. It is essential to schedule routine check-ups with medical professionals in order to evaluate continuing health, modify hormone levels, and handle any new issues. Some who prefer a more laissez-faire attitude to healthcare may see this requirement for continual supervision to be a drawback.

HRT is just one thread in the vast tapestry of perimenopausal choices. Knowing the nuances of its benefits and drawbacks enables one to make an empowered and informed choice that is based on priorities for one's own health as well as goals for a fulfilling life after the hormonal crossroads.

Making Informed Decisions

During the perimenopause, making wise choices is like steering your own ship through unknown waters while maintaining a balance between awareness and confidence. Hormonal swings and physical changes accompany this crucial stage of a woman's life, which calls for a careful and knowledgeable approach.

First and foremost, it becomes critical to understand your body. Hormonal changes coincide with perimenopause, the stage before menopause. Explore the nuances of estrogen and progesterone differences and how they may present in your day-to-day activities. Understanding these subtleties of hormones gives you the power to react to internal changes in an efficient manner.

Armed with this information, it's critical to identify and accept the wide range of possible symptoms. Physical changes frequently take center stage, from hot flashes to irregular menstrual periods. But perimenopause also affects the mind and emotions, exhibiting its effects outside of the body. Developing a customized management strategy for these symptoms begins with acknowledging and embracing them.

Think about how going through perimenopause would affect your general health. Prioritizing physical health is crucial, and changing one's lifestyle is essential. A smoother transition is often aided by specific workout regimens, nutritional methods, and placing a high priority on getting enough sleep. Accepting these aspects strengthens your emotional and mental fortitude in addition to your physical health.

One aspect that is sometimes overlooked during the perimenopause is emotional health. Anxiety, depressive episodes, and mood fluctuations can all become unwanted companions. Effectively managing the emotional rollercoaster requires an understanding of it. Look into coping strategies that work for you, such as mindfulness exercises, asking loved ones for help, or doing enjoyable things.

Relationships may change in the midst of these adjustments. It gets crucial to have open lines of communication with friends, family, and relationships. Bonds are strengthened and understanding is fostered by sharing your experiences. A refined strategy that emphasizes emotional connection and adaptation is also necessary for intimacy.

Although every woman's perimenopausal experience is different, using a comprehensive approach can improve your health. Herbal therapies, mind-body techniques, and integrative medicine provide supplementary forms of care. To guarantee a well-rounded approach, interact with various modalities in accordance with your preferences and seek advice from medical professionals.

For many perimenopausal women, deciding to investigate hormone replacement therapy (HRT) is a critical turning point. Learn about the advantages and disadvantages, balance the risks and potential rewards, and speak with medical professionals. Understanding your unique health profile and balancing it with your comfort level and lifestyle are essential to making an informed decision about HRT.

Enjoy the journey during perimenopause while keeping an eye on the future. Entering menopause is a new beginning rather than an end. Honor the knowledge acquired, the fortitude built, and the self-assurance fostered. Acknowledge aging gracefully and confidently embark on the next phase of your life, equipped with the wisdom to make choices that suit your individual path.

CHAPTER 9: Holistic Approaches to Perimenopausal Health

Integrative Medicine and Perimenopause

As a comprehensive approach to maintaining their well-being, many women are investigating integrative medicine throughout the perimenopause, a time when hormonal changes can feel like a rollercoaster ride. Integrative medicine aims to integrate standard medical procedures with complementary and alternative therapies, rather than to replace them.

Imagine having a toolset that encompasses lifestyle modifications, mind-body techniques, and natural supplements in addition to prescription drugs. That's what integrative medicine is all about, and it's becoming more and more acknowledged as a powerful choice for women figuring out the perimenopause.

Personalized care is a cornerstone of integrative medicine in the perimenopause. Integrative practitioners adopt a holistic approach, taking into account not only physical symptoms but also emotional and spiritual factors, acknowledging that every woman's journey is unique. Instead of just masking symptoms, this method seeks to treat the underlying causes of them.

In integrative medicine, nutrition is crucial during the perimenopause. Some meals have the ability to affect hormone balance and reduce symptoms. Integrative health professionals and nutritionists frequently work together to develop individualized diet regimens that emphasize important nutrients, phytochemicals, and foods that reduce inflammation. It involves providing the body with the proper nutrition to maintain hormonal balance.

Another essential component of integrative medicine is mind-body techniques. Deep breathing exercises, yoga, and mindfulness meditation are some of the techniques that can help women manage stress, get better sleep, and feel better overall. These techniques help women to connect with their bodies during this transition era and also have a calming effect on the nervous system.

Supplements and herbal treatments have a role in the integrative medicine toolbox. Studies have been conducted on the possible advantages of natural compounds such as black cohosh, evening primrose oil, and chaste tree extract in reducing symptoms associated with perimenopause. Although it's important to use caution when taking supplements and speaking with a healthcare provider, many women find relief in the mild assistance that these natural solutions can offer.

Integrative medicine recognizes the psychological and emotional aspects of perimenopause in addition to the physical. Integrative practitioners frequently work in tandem with mental health specialists to provide guidance and assistance in managing emotional fluctuations. This all-encompassing method acknowledges the fundamental connection between physical and mental wellness.

Choosing integrative medicine during the perimenopause is about taking charge of one's health and actively participating in it. It's a synthesis of the greatest ideas from many medical philosophies, addressing the intricacies of this time of life. Upon adopting integrative medicine, women have a greater feeling of agency and a holistic approach that surpasses symptom treatment, promoting a more profound relationship with their bodies and general well-being.

Integrative medicine is a helpful ally in the world of perimenopause, where every woman's experience is as distinct as her fingerprints. It provides a wide range of resources to help women embrace this life-changing stage.

Herbal Remedies and Supplements

Women who are starting the perimenopausal journey frequently look into a variety of natural choices for symptom treatment; among these, herbal medicines and supplements are particularly effective. Imagine them as kind allies on your journey to wellbeing, providing assistance in adjusting to the ups and downs of fluctuating hormone levels.

Herbal Treatments

Many herbs with balancing powers have been bestowed upon us by nature, who is infinitely wise. Of all the green heroes, Black Cohosh is the most prominent. Hot flashes and mood swings can be effectively managed with the help of this herb, which has a reputation for calming the hormonal storm.

Another interesting one is Dong Quai, which is sometimes called the "female ginseng." For generations, this herb has been an essential part of traditional Chinese medicine due to its ability to balance hormones, reduce menstruation discomfort, and soothe other hormonal imbalances. Consider it as a supportive flora companion during the ups and downs of perimenopause.

Support Supplements

Supplements provide an essential supporting role in ensuring your body gets the nutrients it needs, even though herbs are the main attraction. Known as the "sunshine vitamin," vitamin D is crucial for preserving bone health, which is a worry for many women starting this phase of life. Its spotlight moment assists your body in keeping its health and vitality during its everyday dance.

Fish oil supplements provide omega-3 fatty acids, which are great for heart and brain health. Consider them as the silent collaborators in your everyday activities, adding to the well-balanced orchestra of physiological processes.

Discovering Your Own Symphony

Exploring the world of vitamins and herbal therapies is like finding your own special tune for health. Rich in gamma-linolenic acid (GLA), evening primrose oil presents itself as a possible relief for discomfort and soreness in the breasts. It's similar to discovering the ideal note that corresponds with your body's requirements.

It's important to approach these natural partners with knowledge while thinking about them. Speaking with a medical expert guarantees that the decisions you make fit your unique health profile. Your healthcare provider can help you find a harmonious combination of herbal medicines and supplements that are customized to meet your unique needs, much like a conductor conducts an orchestra.

An Orchestra of Caution

Even though there are encouraging signs of alleviation from these nutritional and botanical allies, it's important to use caution and moderation. The key to any music is balance. If you take too many supplements or rely too much on herbal therapies, your body's delicate balance may be upset.

Herbal treatments and dietary supplements are essentially like chapters in your unique wellness narrative. They contribute to a story of wellbeing during the perimenopausal transition by offering depth, color, and support. Accept the voyage with the knowledge of supplementation and the wisdom of nature, and discover a tune that speaks to you personally.

Mind-Body Practices for Well-being

In the complex dance of life, where the body and mind entwine, taking care of both becomes crucial for general health. Adopting mind-body techniques promotes a harmonious balance that flows outward, much like giving a loving embrace to your inner self. Let's investigate the fascinating realm of mind-body techniques, which can serve as your guide through the frequently turbulent perimenopausal years.

1. Mindful Breathing:

Our breathing frequently slips our minds in the rush of everyday life. However, it is the secret to a calm mind. By practicing mindful breathing, you can establish a connection with your breath and become aware of each inhalation and exhalation. This easy exercise calms the inner turmoil and promotes inner serenity by acting as a reset button for your neurological system.

2. Yoga

Yoga is an exquisite tapestry of postures that flow with the breath, a graceful dance between strength and tranquility. You develop mental fortitude as well as physical flexibility as you move through the poses. Yoga's integration of movement and mindfulness is a potent tool for navigating the perimenopause's waves of change, fostering mental and physical well-being.

3. Meditation:

Meditation is the conductor who creates harmony in the mental symphony. You can unravel the strands of stress and anxiety by setting aside a little period of time each day to sit in peaceful contemplation. This practice provides a haven where you can delve into the depths of your thoughts and emotions, promoting a clearer perspective, whether you choose to follow a guided meditation or just concentrate on your breathing.

4. Tai Chi:

Envision a leisurely and elegant dance, with each step blending into the next. That is the core of Tai Chi, a form of martial arts that represents fluidity and balance. Practice of Tai Chi cultivates a profound sense of tranquility in addition to improving physical balance and flexibility. It serves as a gentle reminder to flow with life and with movement.

5. Visualization:

Shut your eyes and picture a calm setting, such a sunny meadow or a peaceful beach. By using visualization, you can paint the canvas of your well-being like an artist would. Traveling inside to a calm place in your mind can be a very effective way to ease tension and encourage relaxation. It's a mental refuge that you can reach at any moment, serving as a private getaway.

6. Progressive Muscle Relaxation:

In the bustle of everyday existence, stress might accompany one for the duration. By methodically tensing and relaxing each muscle group one at a time, Progressive Muscle Relaxation promotes a significant relief of both physical and mental tension. It's a kind of decompression, a subtle reminder that self-care requires letting go.

7. Breathwork:

Breathwork explores deliberate breathing patterns that can revitalize and replenish, going beyond simple conscious breathing. Methods that affect your body's physiological reaction, including diaphragmatic or alternate nostril breathing, can help you relax and regain equilibrium. It's a tune of rebirth for your whole existence, a rhythmic dance with your breath.

Your everyday routine becomes a sanctuary for well-being when you incorporate these mind-body techniques into it. Here, the body and mind move in harmony. Accept these practices as calls to reconnect with yourself, rather than as chores to be completed on a to-do list. This will help you on a path of empowerment and self-discovery during perimenopause and beyond.

CHAPTER 10: Embracing Menopause: Looking Beyond Perimenopause

Transitioning into Menopause

Menopause is like a new chapter in a novel; many women approach this new chapter with a mixture of interest, apprehension, and maybe a hint of nostalgia for bygone days. This phase, which is frequently referred to as a transition, ends the reproductive years and ushers in a time of significant transformations. It includes not just bodily changes but also emotional, social, and psychological ones.

Acknowledging that the menopausal transition is a progressive process rather than an abrupt event is crucial. The years preceding menopause, when hormonal variations cause a variety of physical and emotional changes, are sometimes referred to as the "perimenopause". Accepting this change means realizing that it's an unavoidable and natural phase of a woman's life.

A variety of physiological sensations can result from the drop in progesterone and estrogen levels after menopause. Changes in menstruation patterns, nocturnal sweats, and hot flashes are common companions. Even though these symptoms can be difficult, it's important to keep in mind that each woman's menopausal journey is distinct. It is important to approach this phase with an open mind and a readiness to adjust because what works for one person may not work for another.

Menopause can elicit a range of emotions. Some women experience mood swings and a sense of loss, while others find themselves thinking back on the life they've led thus far. Recognizing these feelings and allowing oneself the grace to work through them is acceptable. During this time of emotional upheaval, getting assistance from friends, family, or even professional counselors can be quite beneficial.

Menopause socially frequently occurs alongside other life transitions. Relationships may be taking on new aspects, occupations may be changing, and children may be leaving the nest. Acknowledging and seizing the opportunities that accompany these shifts is part of accepting menopause. It's an opportunity to take stock of your priorities, explore long-neglected passions, and develop closer relationships with people around you.

Maintaining good physical health is still crucial as menopause approaches. In addition to promoting physical well-being, regular exercise, a healthy diet, and enough sleep assist control the symptoms related to this stage. Accepting menopause means learning to love and respect the body that has supported you through many phases of life, rather than seeing self-care as a luxury.

The wisdom and confidence that typically accompany the menopause transition are among its most amazing features. This is a time to honor the life lessons you've learned and the resiliency that has carried you through successes and setbacks. It's a chance to rethink what it means to be a woman in light of modern standards and expectations, which may have had an impact on earlier periods of existence.

Essentially, entering menopause is a welcome embrace of strength, wisdom, and the ability to choose your own path rather than saying goodbye to youth. Now is the moment to enjoy the voyage and acknowledge that the best parts might still be ahead of you. Therefore, dear woman, as you move through this transformation, remember to treat yourself with love, be receptive to the changes, and celebrate the amazing woman you are growing into.

Embracing Aging with Confidence

It's critical to accept aging with assurance. The theme of this chapter is appreciating the beauty, knowledge, and experience that accrue with age. Now let's get started and see how you can move through this stage with confidence and grace.

Let's start by dispelling the misconception that becoming older means being less valuable or appealing. On the contrary! You have the chance to define beauty according to your own standards during your perimenopause journey. Those sentences about laughing? They serve as a monument to a happy, full life full with innumerable tales. Accept them as honorifics rather than indicators of aging.

Recall that confidence comes from the inside out as your physique transforms. Put your attention on taking care of your physical health in a way that makes you feel good. Find activities that help you feel more connected to your body and confident in yourself, whether it's a vigorous walk, a yoga session, or even just dancing around your living room (yes, please feel free to dance if you enjoy it!).

In reference to self-worth, let's discuss the psychological and affective dimensions of accepting aging. There are times when mood swings and an emotional rollercoaster accompany perimenopause. It's critical to stay optimistic and to recognize and respect these emotions. Make sure you have a strong support system of friends and family that encourage you, and don't be afraid to ask for expert assistance when necessary.

Let's talk about the enchanted word now: self-love. It's a potent practice, not simply a catchphrase. The first step to confidently accepting aging is to fully accept who you are. Every day, set aside some time to celebrate the amazing woman you are on the inside and out. Remind yourself that self-love is a journey rather than a destination, show yourself kindness, and engage in enjoyable activities.

Evaluate your objectives and desires as you move through the perimenopause. Now is the perfect moment to revisit hobbies and passions that you may have neglected in the rush of previous years. Take advantage of the chance to reevaluate your objectives and forge a rewarding route for this new stage of life, whether it's picking up a new skill, beginning a hobby, or taking on a long-desired project.

Let's discuss style and fashion as well. Accepting your age also implies accepting your changing sense of style. Add items to your wardrobe that give you a sense of comfort and confidence. Play around with hues, materials, and fashions to showcase the colorful, individual lady you are. Your clothing choices can be a strong statement of your originality and confidence.

Recall that confidence is an infectious mental attitude. Embrace the good people in your life and partake in inspiring and motivating activities. Look for role models who have confidently and gracefully aged; their experiences might serve as inspiration for your own journey.

In conclusion, it's important to celebrate the amazing person you've become, maintain your wellbeing, and accept aging with confidence during perimenopause. This stage is a welcome embracing of the rich, rewarding chapters that lie ahead rather than a farewell to youth. You are a force to be reckoned with, my friend—beautiful, wise, and all around amazing! So go forward with confidence!

Celebrating the Next Chapter of Life

Starting a new chapter in life is like walking onto a stage that is full of opportunities, learning opportunities, and the beauty of development. Menopause is upon us, and we should celebrate, take stock of our lives, and look forward to what is ahead as we bid the perimenopausal phase goodnight.

Amid the hormonal upheavals and changes that accompany perimenopause, it's natural to feel overwhelmed and maybe even a little nervous about what's ahead. But rather than just coming to an end, this stage is a gateway to something new. Let's explore the reasons why it's not only necessary but also a decision to celebrate the start of a new chapter in life.

A crucial element of this festivity involves recognizing the fortitude and tenacity that have propelled you so far. The ups and downs of the perimenopause are a tribute to your ability to adjust and flourish. Give yourself a minute to reflect on the woman you have grown into: one who is more self-aware, wiser, and prepared for the adventures that lie ahead.

There is a special sense of release that comes with entering menopause. Menstrual cycle endings don't mean life is coming to an end; rather, they herald a new chapter in the story of femininity. Breaking free from the monthly cycle of menstruation can lead to a renewed sense of autonomy and an opportunity to focus energy on activities that fulfill and offer happiness.

Menopause is also a good time to review and reshape personal objectives. Think of it as an opportunity to explore interests that might have been neglected during the busy years spent developing a profession or raising children. You can write the next chapter by rekindling your creative spark, taking up a new pastime, or going on a long-awaited journey.

Celebrating the next chapter involves more than just personal development; it also entails fostering bonds with others and forging deeper ties. Menopause may present a chance to deepen relationships with friends, partners, and children as it frequently corresponds with changes in family dynamics. Open dialogue regarding this period of transition can promote empathy and support, laying the groundwork for life experiences and good humor.

Menopause brings with it physical changes, but it also presents an opportunity to develop a healthy relationship with your body. Adopting a self-care mindset entails appreciating the changes as well as accepting them. Celebrate the strength that has helped you get through a variety of life situations, the wisdom that comes with age, and the lines of laughter that tell tales of delight.

This chapter also serves as a blank canvas for creativity. Adopt new hobbies, push yourself with novel viewpoints, and let go of any stereotypes about getting older. As women get older, society frequently imposes restrictive preconceptions on them. However, now is the ideal moment to challenge these notions and redefine what it means to be a vibrant, self-assured, and powerful woman.

It's important to recognize that self-care goes beyond maintaining one's physical health when we celebrate the beginning of a new chapter in life. Maintaining emotional and mental well-being is equally important. Spend some time reflecting, practice mindfulness, and surround yourself with understanding and supportive people. This chapter is about accepting all aspects of your multifaceted self and living a holistic life.

To sum up, marking the beginning of a new chapter in your life is a pledge to cherish the abundance of what lies ahead as well as an acknowledgement of the amazing journey you have already taken. It's about having the courage to dream and succeed beyond social norms, welcoming change with open arms, and basking in newly discovered freedom. Here's to you, then—to the beauty, courage, and knowledge that characterize this incredible phase of your life. I hope it is full of happiness, contentment, and the steadfast conviction that the best is still to come.